Fit After 40: The Ultimate Nutritional Guide for Men

By
Dr. C. Shawn

Tom (Age 40)

I've struggled with maintaining my fitness since turning 40, but this book has given me the tools I needed. The meal plans are tailored to our age group, and the emphasis on balanced nutrition has helped me regain muscle and lose stubborn fat.

Ryan (Age 42)

This book is a gem for men like me who want to make lasting changes to their health. It's informative without being overwhelming, and the meal plans are realistic and sustainable. I'm on track to achieving my weight loss and muscle gain goals thanks to the guidance within these pages.

Carlos (Age 42)

I can't believe this book, it's a total game-changer! The food plans are simple, and they're helping me drop pounds like nobody's business. Feeling stronger and loving the vibes!

Jamal (Age 45)

Let me tell you, this book is a straight-up blessing. The meal ideas are mad tasty, and I'm seeing the scale drop. It's like having a secret weapon for getting fit.

David (Age 48)

Man, this book is gold. It's breaking down all the food stuff in a way I can actually understand. I'm lighter on my feet, and it's like I've got a new lease on life.

Chapter List:

1. **The Changing Landscape: Men's Health After 40**

2. **Understanding Nutritional Needs: A Deep Dive**

3. **Crafting Your 30-Day Meal Plan: A Step-by-Step Approach**

4. **Grocery Shopping Made Effective and Easy**

5. **Cooking for Success: Recipes Tailored for Men Over 40**

6. **The Power of Protein: Building and Maintaining Muscle Mass**

7. **The Role of Carbohydrates: Fuelling Your Active Lifestyle**

8. **Fats Unveiled: Making Smart Choices for Heart Health**

9. **Micronutrients and Antioxidants: Essential Elements for Longevity**

10. **Hydration and Its Impact on Overall Fitness**

11. **Pre-Workout and Post-Workout Nutrition: Optimizing Your Routine**

12. **Managing Metabolism: Diet's Influence on Weight Loss**

13. **Overcoming Challenges: From Cravings to Social Situations**

Introduction:

Embarking on a journey towards better health and fitness after the age of 40 might seem like a daunting task, but it's a venture that holds tremendous promise. "Fit After 40: The Ultimate Nutritional Guide for Men" is your comprehensive companion in this transformative journey. This book is not just about losing weight and gaining muscle; it's about embracing a healthier lifestyle that extends beyond physical appearance, enhancing your overall well-being and vitality.

With age, our bodies undergo various changes that impact how we process and utilize nutrients. Hormonal shifts, slowed metabolism, and changing activity levels all play a role in determining the dietary needs of men over 40. This book aims to unravel the complexities of nutrition during this phase of life, providing you with a science-backed, practical roadmap to revitalize your health.

Chapter 1: The Changing Landscape: Men's Health After 40
As men cross the threshold of 40, they often notice shifts in their energy levels, muscle mass, and overall vitality. In this chapter, we delve into the biological changes that accompany this phase of life. From the decline in testosterone levels to the gradual decrease in metabolic rate, understanding these shifts forms the foundation of making informed nutritional choices. We also address common concerns such as weight gain, joint health, and cardiovascular risk, setting the stage for a targeted approach to dietary adjustments.

Chapter 2: Understanding Nutritional Needs: A Deep Dive
Nutrition is not a one-size-fits-all concept, and this truth becomes even more evident after 40. In this chapter, we explore the intricate interplay of macronutrients and micronutrients in the

context of men's health. Protein's role in muscle maintenance and repair, carbohydrates as fuel for physical activity, and the significance of healthy fats are all examined in detail. Additionally, we unravel the mystery of micronutrients and their impact on immune function and longevity.

Chapter 3: Crafting Your 30-Day Meal Plan: A Step-by-Step Approach

The key to sustained change lies in planning. In this chapter, we guide you through the process of creating a personalized 30-day meal plan. We take into account your individual goals, activity levels, and dietary preferences. From calculating your daily caloric needs to distributing macronutrients across meals, this step-by-step approach ensures that your nutrition aligns with your objectives.

Chapter 4: Grocery Shopping Made Effective and Easy

Navigating the aisles of the grocery store can be overwhelming, but armed with the right knowledge, it becomes a breeze. Chapter 4 equips you with the skills to make smart choices while shopping for fresh produce, lean proteins, whole grains, and nutrient-dense snacks. We provide tips on reading food labels, identifying hidden sugars and additives, and choosing organic options when necessary.

Chapter 5: Cooking for Success: Recipes Tailored for Men Over 40

Healthy eating doesn't mean sacrificing flavor. In fact, it's an opportunity to explore new culinary horizons. This chapter presents a collection of recipes designed to cater to the nutritional needs of men over 40. From hearty breakfast options to satisfying dinners, these recipes are both delicious and nutrient-packed. We also offer cooking tips and meal prep strategies to make healthy eating a seamless part of your routine.

Chapter 6: The Power of Protein: Building and Maintaining Muscle Mass

Muscle loss is a common concern as men age, but it's not an inevitability. Protein, often referred to as the building block of muscles, plays a pivotal role in preserving and even increasing muscle mass. This chapter delves into the optimal protein intake for men over 40, the importance of amino acids, and sources of high-quality protein. We also address myths surrounding protein supplementation and highlight the significance of timing protein intake around workouts.

Chapter 7: The Role of Carbohydrates: Fuelling Your Active Lifestyle

Carbohydrates are the body's primary source of energy, making them crucial for maintaining an active lifestyle. In this chapter, we discuss the different types of carbohydrates, their glycemic impact, and how to strike a balance between energy intake and expenditure. Whether you're an avid athlete or simply looking to stay active, understanding carbohydrate utilization can help you optimize your performance and recovery.

Chapter 8: Fats Unveiled: Making Smart Choices for Heart Health

The relationship between dietary fat and heart health has long been debated. In this chapter, we unravel the complexities surrounding fats, from saturated to unsaturated varieties. By understanding the impact of fats on cholesterol levels and inflammation, you can make informed choices that promote cardiovascular well-being. We also explore sources of healthy fats and offer guidance on incorporating them into your diet.

Chapter 9: Micronutrients and Antioxidants: Essential Elements for Longevity

Vitamins, minerals, and antioxidants are the unsung heroes of optimal health. Chapter 9 explores the role of these micronutrients in supporting immune function, cellular repair, and disease prevention. We highlight specific micronutrients that hold particular importance for men over 40 and provide a roadmap to ensure you're meeting your body's requirements through your diet and, if necessary, supplementation.

Chapter 10: Hydration and Its Impact on Overall Fitness

Staying adequately hydrated is often overlooked but is essential for overall well-being. In this chapter, we dive into the importance of hydration for cognitive function, digestion, and physical performance. We provide guidelines for estimating your fluid needs, tips for incorporating hydrating foods into your diet, and strategies for maintaining proper hydration throughout the day.

Chapter 11: Pre-Workout and Post-Workout Nutrition: Optimizing Your Routine

Fueling your body before and after exercise can greatly impact your workout performance and recovery. Chapter 11 discusses the ideal pre-workout meal composition to enhance energy levels and endurance. Additionally, we explore post-workout nutrition, including the importance of protein and carbohydrates in promoting muscle recovery and growth.

Chapter 12: Managing Metabolism: Diet's Influence on Weight Loss

Metabolism tends to slow down with age, but the right dietary strategies can help you manage your weight effectively. This chapter delves into the science of metabolism and the role of calories in weight management. We discuss how to create a calorie deficit through diet while ensuring you're still receiving essential nutrients. Practical tips for overcoming weight loss plateaus are also provided.

Chapter 13: Overcoming Challenges: From Cravings to Social Situations
No health journey is without its challenges. Chapter 13 addresses common obstacles such as cravings, emotional eating, and navigating social situations. Strategies to curb cravings, manage stress-related eating, and make healthy choices when dining out are all covered in this chapter. By developing a resilient mindset and arming yourself with coping strategies, you can stay on track even when faced with temptations.

Chapter 14: Sustainable Habits: Turning Nutrition into a Lifestyle
Achieving your health goals is not a sprint; it's a marathon. Sustainable habits are the cornerstone of long-term success. In this chapter, we discuss the importance of consistency and how to transform healthy eating practices into a sustainable lifestyle. We delve into meal planning hacks, mindful eating techniques, and strategies for maintaining motivation over the long haul.

Chapter 15: Staying on Track: Strategies for Long-Term Success
As you wrap up your journey through "Fit After 40," Chapter 15 provides you with a comprehensive toolkit for maintaining the progress you've made. We explore monitoring techniques, ways to adjust your meal plan as your goals evolve, and strategies to prevent relapses. Additionally, we emphasize the connection between nutrition, exercise, and holistic well-being.

"Fit After 40: The Ultimate Nutritional Guide for Men" is more than just a book; it's your partner in revitalizing your health, improving your fitness, and enhancing your quality of life. With science-based insights, practical tips, and a holistic approach to nutrition, this guide empowers you to take control of your well-being and embrace a vibrant future after 40. Your journey towards a healthier, stronger, and more energized you starts now.

Chapter 1: The Changing Landscape: Men's Health After 40

The journey of life is marked by transitions, and one of the most significant transitions occurs as men step into their 40s. This pivotal period is characterized by a series of physiological and hormonal changes that can impact various aspects of men's health. "The Changing Landscape: Men's Health After 40" takes a deep dive into these transformations, exploring how they affect everything from energy levels to muscle mass, and providing valuable insights into navigating this new chapter of life.

Biological Shifts and Hormonal Changes:
As men age, their bodies undergo a series of biological shifts that can influence their health and well-being. One of the most notable changes is a decline in testosterone levels. Testosterone, often referred to as the "male hormone," plays a crucial role in muscle development, bone density, and overall vitality. Its decline can lead to decreased muscle mass, lower energy levels, and even changes in mood and cognition.

Moreover, metabolic rate tends to slow down with age. This means that the body burns calories at a slower pace, making weight management more challenging. This slowdown can be attributed to a decrease in muscle mass, as muscles are more metabolically active than fat tissue. As a result, men might find that they gain weight more easily and struggle to shed excess pounds.

Weight Gain and Cardiovascular Health:
Weight gain, particularly around the midsection, is a common concern for men over 40. This increase in abdominal fat is not

solely an aesthetic issue; it also has implications for cardiovascular health. Belly fat, also known as visceral fat, is associated with an increased risk of heart disease, diabetes, and other metabolic disorders. This is because visceral fat is metabolically active and can release inflammatory molecules that contribute to chronic diseases.

Furthermore, cardiovascular health becomes an important focus after 40. The risk of conditions like high blood pressure, cholesterol imbalances, and heart disease tends to rise with age. Lifestyle factors, including diet and exercise, play a crucial role in mitigating these risks. Understanding how dietary choices can impact cardiovascular health becomes essential for promoting longevity and vitality.

Joint Health and Bone Density:
The wear and tear of life become more evident in joint health as men enter their 40s. Joints may become stiffer and less flexible, and conditions like arthritis can become more prevalent. Proper nutrition and exercise play a significant role in supporting joint health, ensuring that the body remains mobile and functional.

Bone density is another aspect that undergoes changes with age. While osteoporosis is often associated with women, men are also at risk of developing this condition. As bone density decreases, the risk of fractures and injuries increases. Adequate calcium and vitamin D intake, along with weight-bearing exercises, are vital for maintaining strong bones.

Cognitive Function and Mental Health:
Cognitive changes are part of the aging process, but they can be exacerbated by other factors. Hormonal shifts, particularly the decline in testosterone, can impact cognitive function. Men might notice changes in memory, focus, and even mood. It's

crucial to recognize these changes and adopt strategies to support cognitive health, such as engaging in mentally stimulating activities and maintaining a balanced diet.

Mental health is another significant consideration. While mental health issues are not exclusive to any age group, they can manifest differently in men over 40. Depression, anxiety, and stress can be influenced by hormonal changes, lifestyle factors, and the challenges that come with midlife transitions. Nurturing mental well-being through proper nutrition and seeking professional support when needed is essential.

Embracing Change and Wellness:
"The Changing Landscape: Men's Health After 40" emphasizes the importance of embracing change and proactively addressing the shifts that come with age. While these changes are natural, they don't have to signify a decline in well-being. With the right knowledge and strategies, men can navigate this new phase of life with vitality and resilience.

Understanding the hormonal shifts, metabolic changes, and their impacts on weight, cardiovascular health, joint health, bone density, cognitive function, and mental well-being is the first step towards making informed choices. By recognizing that wellness is a multifaceted journey encompassing physical, mental, and emotional aspects, men can take charge of their health after 40 and embark on a path of empowerment, longevity, and overall well-being.

Chapter 2: Understanding Nutritional Needs: A Deep Dive

Nutrition is the foundation of health and well-being, and its importance becomes even more pronounced as men step into their 40s. "Understanding Nutritional Needs: A Deep Dive" delves into the intricate interplay of nutrients, their roles in the body, and how they evolve with age. This chapter aims to provide a comprehensive understanding of the macronutrients and micronutrients that contribute to optimal health for men over 40.

Macronutrients: Fuel for the Body

Macronutrients are the essential components of our diet that provide energy and support various bodily functions. These include carbohydrates, proteins, and fats, each with its distinct role in maintaining health.

Carbohydrates:
Carbohydrates are the body's primary source of energy, particularly for brain function and physical activity. However, the types of carbohydrates consumed can significantly impact health. Simple carbohydrates, found in sugary snacks and refined grains, can lead to rapid spikes and crashes in blood sugar levels. This can be problematic for men over 40, as unstable blood sugar levels are linked to increased risk of diabetes, weight gain, and energy fluctuations.

Complex carbohydrates, on the other hand, are found in whole grains, vegetables, and legumes. They provide a steady release of energy and are rich in fiber, which supports digestive health and helps regulate blood sugar levels. For men over 40, incorporating complex carbohydrates into their diet can aid in maintaining stable energy levels and promoting overall health.

Proteins:
Proteins are the building blocks of the body, essential for the repair and maintenance of tissues, muscles, and enzymes. As men age, maintaining muscle mass becomes increasingly important. Protein intake plays a critical role in this process, as a decline in muscle mass can lead to decreased metabolism and overall functional decline.

Adequate protein intake also supports immune function, hormone production, and the synthesis of neurotransmitters that regulate mood and cognition. Men over 40 should focus on including lean sources of protein such as poultry, fish, lean meats, eggs, dairy products, and plant-based options like legumes and tofu. Distributing protein intake evenly across meals can help optimize muscle protein synthesis throughout the day.

Fats:
Dietary fat is often misunderstood, but it's a crucial component of health. Fats provide concentrated energy, support cell structure, and aid in the absorption of fat-soluble vitamins (A, D, E, and K). For men over 40, heart health becomes a priority, and the quality of fats consumed plays a pivotal role in this regard.

Healthy fats, such as monounsaturated and polyunsaturated fats, found in olive oil, nuts, seeds, and fatty fish, have been associated with a reduced risk of heart disease. These fats help lower bad cholesterol levels, decrease inflammation, and promote overall cardiovascular well-being. Saturated fats and trans fats, often found in processed foods and fried items, should be limited as they can raise bad cholesterol levels and increase the risk of heart disease.

Micronutrients: The Guardians of Health

Micronutrients are vitamins and minerals that the body requires in smaller quantities but are essential for numerous physiological processes.

Vitamins and Minerals:
Vitamins and minerals act as co-factors in enzymatic reactions, support immune function, aid in energy production, and contribute to overall health. For men over 40, specific micronutrients take on increased importance.

Vitamin D, often referred to as the "sunshine vitamin," is crucial for bone health as it aids in calcium absorption. As bone density becomes a concern with age, ensuring adequate vitamin D intake is vital.

Vitamin B12 is essential for nerve function and the production of red blood cells. With age, the body's ability to absorb vitamin B12 from food sources may decrease, making supplementation or consumption of fortified foods important.

Calcium is essential for maintaining strong bones and preventing osteoporosis. It's not just about dairy; incorporating leafy greens, fortified plant-based milk, and other calcium-rich foods is essential.

Antioxidants, such as vitamins C and E, along with minerals like selenium and zinc, play a role in neutralizing free radicals that can damage cells and contribute to aging. Ensuring a diet rich in fruits, vegetables, nuts, and whole grains provides the body with a variety of antioxidants.

Hydration: The Unsung Hero

Water, often overlooked, is a fundamental component of nutrition. Staying adequately hydrated is crucial for digestion, nutrient transport, temperature regulation, and overall bodily functions. As men age, the sense of thirst may become less acute, making it important to consciously monitor fluid intake.

Proper hydration supports joint health, cognitive function, and digestion, and can even aid in weight management by promoting satiety. Men over 40 should aim to drink plenty of water throughout the day and consider hydrating foods like fruits and vegetables as part of their diet.

Personalization and Balance: The Key to Nutritional Success

"Understanding Nutritional Needs: A Deep Dive" underscores the importance of personalized nutrition. Men over 40 have unique dietary requirements influenced by their activity levels, health goals, and individual metabolic rates. A balanced approach that includes a variety of whole foods from different macronutrient and micronutrient sources is the cornerstone of optimal health.

By comprehending the intricate roles of macronutrients and micronutrients in the body, men can make informed choices that empower them to age gracefully, maintain energy levels, preserve muscle mass, support heart health, and enhance overall well-being. This deep dive into nutrition serves as a roadmap for building a strong foundation of health that will carry men through their 40s and beyond, ensuring they enjoy vitality and quality of life at every stage.

Chapter 3: Crafting Your 30-Day Meal Plan: A Step-by-Step Approach

In the pursuit of optimal health and well-being, a well-structured meal plan is a powerful tool. "Crafting Your 30-Day Meal Plan: A Step-by-Step Approach" dives into the process of creating a personalized and sustainable meal plan tailored to the specific nutritional needs of men over 40. This chapter aims to guide you through the intricate process of designing meals that support your goals, accommodate your lifestyle, and foster a healthier relationship with food.

Setting the Stage: Define Your Goals

The first step in crafting your 30-day meal plan is to define your goals. Are you aiming to lose weight, gain muscle, enhance energy levels, or simply improve overall health? Clarity in your objectives will guide the composition of your meal plan. For example, if muscle gain is a priority, protein intake and portion sizes will be crucial considerations.

Calculate Your Caloric Needs: A Foundation for Planning

Understanding your caloric needs is essential to create a meal plan that supports your goals without overindulging or undernourishing yourself. Online calculators or consulting a nutritionist can help estimate your daily caloric requirements based on factors like age, activity level, and goals.

Distribute Macronutrients: Balancing Proteins, Carbs, and Fats

Once you have your daily caloric target, the next step is to distribute macronutrients – proteins, carbohydrates, and fats –

in a balanced manner. Proteins are crucial for muscle health, carbohydrates provide energy, and fats support overall bodily functions.

A common approach is the macronutrient split: around 30% of calories from proteins, 40% from carbohydrates, and 30% from healthy fats. Adjustments can be made based on personal preferences, activity levels, and goals. For instance, if you're more active, you might need slightly more carbohydrates to fuel your workouts.

Creating Balanced Meals: The Plate Method

The plate method is a simple and effective way to structure your meals. Visualize your plate divided into sections: half for vegetables and fruits, one-quarter for lean proteins, and one-quarter for whole grains or starchy vegetables. This method ensures a balanced intake of nutrients while controlling portion sizes.

Variety and Nutrient Density: A Rainbow of Foods

Variety is the spice of life, especially in your diet. Different foods offer different nutrients, so a diverse range of fruits, vegetables, whole grains, lean proteins, and healthy fats should be included. "Eating the rainbow" ensures you're getting a spectrum of vitamins, minerals, and antioxidants.

Meal Timing and Frequency: Nourishing Consistency

The timing of your meals can impact energy levels, metabolism, and overall digestion. Aim for regular meal times to maintain steady blood sugar levels and prevent overeating due to excessive hunger. Space out your meals to include three main meals and two to three snacks, depending on your activity level.

Plan Ahead: Weekly Meal Prepping

Meal prepping is a game-changer when it comes to sticking to a healthy eating plan. Dedicate time each week to prepare ingredients, cook meals, and portion them into containers. This not only saves time but also prevents impulsive and unhealthy food choices when you're pressed for time or hungry.

Flexibility and Enjoyment: Including Your Favorites

A balanced meal plan doesn't mean deprivation. It's essential to include foods you love to maintain a healthy relationship with food. Incorporate your favorite dishes or treats in moderation to prevent feelings of restriction and enhance long-term adherence.

Monitor and Adjust: Listening to Your Body

Your meal plan is a living document. Regularly monitor how your body responds to different foods and portion sizes. Energy levels, mood, digestion, and progress toward your goals are all important indicators. If needed, make adjustments to your meal plan based on these cues.

Mindful Eating: Savoring Every Bite

Beyond the science of nutrition, the practice of mindful eating adds depth to your meal plan. Pay attention to your body's hunger and fullness cues, chew slowly, and savor the flavors.

Mindful eating fosters a better connection with your body and can prevent overeating.

Staying Hydrated: The Unsung Hero

Water is often overlooked but plays a vital role in overall health. Adequate hydration supports digestion, cognitive function, and energy levels. Incorporate water-rich foods like fruits and vegetables and aim to drink plenty of water throughout the day.

Embrace Progress, Not Perfection

"Crafting Your 30-Day Meal Plan: A Step-by-Step Approach" emphasizes the importance of a holistic and individualized approach to meal planning. While structure is essential, flexibility, enjoyment, and self-compassion are equally vital. Your meal plan is a tool to support your goals, but it should also enhance your quality of life. As you embark on this journey, remember that progress, not perfection, is the ultimate goal. Through mindful planning, balanced choices, and self-awareness, you're well on your way to crafting a sustainable and nourishing meal plan that will fuel your health and vitality for years to come.

Chapter 4: Grocery Shopping Made Effective and Easy

Grocery shopping forms the foundation of a healthy eating plan. "Grocery Shopping Made Effective and Easy" guides you through the art of smart grocery shopping, ensuring that your kitchen is stocked with nutrient-rich foods that support your health goals. This chapter unveils strategies to navigate the aisles, read food labels, make informed choices, and transform your grocery shopping experience into a seamless and empowering endeavor.

Planning Before You Go: The Key to Success

Effective grocery shopping starts before you even step foot in the store. Taking time to plan your meals for the week and create a detailed shopping list is crucial. Plan your breakfasts, lunches, dinners, and snacks, and jot down the ingredients you'll need. This prevents impulsive purchases and helps you stick to your meal plan.

Navigating the Aisles: Staying Focused

Grocery stores can be overwhelming with their aisles packed with a myriad of choices. To stay focused and on track, shop the perimeter of the store first. This is where you'll find fresh produce, lean proteins, dairy, and whole grains. The center aisles often house processed and packaged foods, so approach them with caution.

Reading Food Labels: Decoding Nutritional Information

Food labels provide a wealth of information, but they can also be confusing. Start by checking the serving size – it's easy to underestimate portions. Look for the total calories, as well as the breakdown of macronutrients (proteins, carbohydrates, fats). Pay attention to added sugars and sodium content, as excessive consumption of these can have negative health impacts.

Choosing Fresh Produce: Opt for Colorful Variety

Aim to fill your cart with an array of colorful fruits and vegetables. Different colors indicate varying nutrient profiles. For instance, orange and dark leafy greens are rich in vitamins A and C, while berries boast antioxidants. Fresh produce provides essential vitamins, minerals, fiber, and antioxidants that support overall health.

Navigating the Meat and Seafood Section: Prioritize Lean Protein

When selecting meats, opt for lean cuts to reduce saturated fat intake. Look for skinless poultry, lean cuts of beef, and pork with minimal visible fat. Seafood, particularly fatty fish like salmon, mackerel, and sardines, provide omega-3 fatty acids that are beneficial for heart health and inflammation.

The Dairy Aisle: Choosing Wisely

In the dairy aisle, choose low-fat or fat-free options. Greek yogurt is a protein-rich choice, and unsweetened almond or soy milk are great alternatives to dairy milk. When selecting cheese, opt for reduced-fat or part-skim varieties.

Navigating the Grain Aisle: Whole Grains Are Key

Whole grains are a staple of a healthy diet. Look for whole wheat, quinoa, brown rice, and oats. Avoid refined grains that lack fiber and nutrients. Whole grains provide sustained energy, fiber, and essential nutrients.

Canned Goods and Frozen Foods: Check for Nutrient Density

Canned goods and frozen foods can be convenient, but they vary in nutritional quality. Choose canned goods with no added sugars and low sodium options. For frozen fruits and vegetables, opt for those without added sauces or seasonings. These options can be just as nutritious as fresh produce.

Staying Mindful in the Snack Aisle: Opt for Nutrient-Rich Snacks

Snack choices are important. Choose snacks that provide nutritional value rather than empty calories. Nuts, seeds, whole-grain crackers, and fresh fruit are excellent choices. Be cautious with pre-packaged snacks, as they can be high in added sugars, sodium, and unhealthy fats.

Checking Out: Last-Minute Considerations

As you approach the checkout, take a final look at your cart. Did you cover all the major food groups? Is your cart filled with whole foods and minimally processed items? Remember, every item you place in your cart contributes to your overall health.

Empowering Your Choices

"Grocery Shopping Made Effective and Easy" is more than a mundane chore – it's an opportunity to nourish your body and make choices that support your well-being. By planning your meals, understanding food labels, and prioritizing fresh, nutrient-dense foods, you're taking significant steps toward achieving your health goals. As you embark on this journey, remember that each grocery trip is a chance to empower yourself with knowledge, make informed decisions, and cultivate a positive relationship with the foods that fuel your vitality and longevity.

Chapter 5: Cooking for Success: Recipes Tailored for Men Over 40

The kitchen is where your healthy meal plans come to life. "Cooking for Success: Recipes Tailored for Men Over 40" takes you on a culinary journey, offering a collection of nutrient-packed recipes designed to cater to the specific nutritional needs of men entering this transformative phase of life. From hearty breakfasts to satisfying dinners, these recipes are not only delicious but also contribute to your overall well-being.

The Power of a Nutrient-Rich Breakfast:

Recipe: Protein-Packed Breakfast Bowl
- Ingredients:
  - 1/2 cup cooked quinoa
  - 1/4 cup Greek yogurt
  - 1/4 cup mixed berries
  - 1 tablespoon chopped nuts (almonds, walnuts)
  - 1 tablespoon chia seeds
  - 1 teaspoon honey (optional)
- Instructions:
  - In a bowl, layer cooked quinoa, Greek yogurt, and mixed berries.
  - Top with chopped nuts, chia seeds, and a drizzle of honey if desired.
  - This breakfast bowl is rich in protein, fiber, and healthy fats, providing sustained energy and supporting muscle health.

Balanced Lunches for Sustained Energy:

Recipe: Grilled Chicken and Quinoa Salad
- Ingredients:

  - 4 oz grilled chicken breast, sliced
  - 1 cup cooked quinoa
  - 2 cups mixed salad greens
  - 1/4 cup cherry tomatoes, halved
  - 1/4 cucumber, sliced
  - 2 tablespoons feta cheese
  - 1 tablespoon balsamic vinaigrette
- Instructions:
  - Arrange salad greens on a plate and top with cooked quinoa.
  - Add grilled chicken, cherry tomatoes, cucumber, and feta cheese.
  - Drizzle with balsamic vinaigrette for a balanced and flavorful lunch.

Energizing Snacks to Fuel Your Day:

Recipe: Nut Butter and Apple Slices
- Ingredients:
  - 1 apple, sliced
  - 2 tablespoons nut butter (almond, peanut, or cashew)
- Instructions:
  - Slice the apple into wedges.
  - Dip apple slices in your choice of nut butter for a satisfying snack rich in fiber, healthy fats, and a hint of sweetness.

Dinner Delights for Nourishment:

Recipe: Baked Salmon with Roasted Vegetables
- Ingredients:
  - 6 oz salmon fillet
  - 1 cup mixed vegetables (broccoli, carrots, bell peppers)
  - 1 tablespoon olive oil
  - 1 teaspoon lemon juice
  - Fresh herbs (rosemary, thyme)

- Instructions:
  - Preheat the oven to 400°F (200°C).
  - Toss mixed vegetables with olive oil, lemon juice, and fresh herbs.
  - Place salmon fillet on a baking sheet and surround with vegetables.
  - Bake for 15-20 minutes, until salmon is cooked through and vegetables are tender.
  - This recipe provides omega-3 fatty acids, protein, and a variety of vitamins and minerals.

Creating Balanced Snacks:

Recipe: Greek Yogurt Parfait
- Ingredients:
  - 1/2 cup Greek yogurt
  - 1/4 cup granola (choose a low-sugar option)
  - 1/4 cup mixed berries
  - 1 tablespoon chopped nuts
- Instructions:
  - In a glass or bowl, layer Greek yogurt, granola, mixed berries, and chopped nuts.
  - This parfait is rich in protein, probiotics, and antioxidants, making it a satisfying and nutritious snack.

Indulging in Healthy Desserts:

Recipe: Dark Chocolate-Dipped Strawberries
- Ingredients:
  - 6-8 fresh strawberries
  - 1 oz dark chocolate (70% cocoa or higher)
- Instructions:
  - Melt dark chocolate using a double boiler or microwave.

- Dip each strawberry into the melted chocolate, allowing excess to drip off.
   - Place strawberries on parchment paper and refrigerate until chocolate hardens.
   - Dark chocolate provides antioxidants, and strawberries offer vitamins and fiber, creating a guilt-free dessert option.

The Art of Meal Prepping:

Recipe: Quinoa and Vegetable Stir-Fry
- Ingredients:
   - 1 cup cooked quinoa
   - 1 cup mixed vegetables (bell peppers, snap peas, carrots)
   - 4 oz cooked chicken or tofu
   - 2 tablespoons low-sodium soy sauce
   - 1 teaspoon sesame oil
   - 1 teaspoon minced garlic
- Instructions:
   - In a skillet, heat sesame oil and minced garlic.
   - Add mixed vegetables and sauté until tender.
   - Stir in cooked quinoa, cooked chicken or tofu, and soy sauce.
   - Toss until everything is heated through and well combined.
   - This stir-fry is a balanced meal that can be prepared in advance and reheated for a quick and nutritious dinner.

Nourishing Through Every Bite

"Cooking for Success: Recipes Tailored for Men Over 40" elevates your culinary experience, making the journey toward health and vitality an enjoyable one. These recipes combine flavors, textures, and nutrients to create meals that nourish your body and delight your taste buds. From breakfasts that provide sustained energy to balanced lunches, energizing snacks, and satisfying dinners, each recipe is designed to support your goals and overall well-being. As you step into the kitchen and explore these dishes, remember that every meal is an opportunity to invest in your health, take control of your nutrition, and embrace a vibrant future after 40.

<u>Chapter 6: The Power of Protein: Building and Maintaining Muscle Mass</u>

Muscle mass is not just about appearance; it plays a crucial role in overall health, mobility, and vitality. "The Power of Protein: Building and Maintaining Muscle Mass" delves into the science of protein, exploring its significance in maintaining muscle health as men progress beyond 40. This chapter unveils strategies to optimize protein intake, enhance muscle growth, and ensure that your body remains strong, functional, and resilient.

Understanding Muscle Health: The Importance of Muscle Mass

Muscle mass is a dynamic and metabolically active tissue that contributes to numerous bodily functions. Beyond movement, muscles play a role in metabolic regulation, blood sugar control, and even immune function. As men age, maintaining muscle mass becomes increasingly important, as the natural decline in testosterone and physical activity can lead to muscle loss, a condition known as sarcopenia.

The Role of Protein: Fueling Muscle Growth and Repair

Protein is often hailed as the building block of muscle, and rightfully so. Proteins are composed of amino acids, which are essential for muscle repair, growth, and maintenance. When you engage in physical activity, especially resistance training, you create microtears in your muscles. Adequate protein intake provides the amino acids needed to repair and strengthen these muscles, promoting muscle growth over time.

Protein Requirements: Tailoring Intake to Your Goals

Protein needs can vary based on factors like age, activity level, and fitness goals. Men over 40, especially those aiming to maintain or increase muscle mass, should pay attention to their protein intake. A general guideline is to aim for around 1.2 to 1.5 grams of protein per kilogram of body weight per day. For instance, a 70 kg (154 lb) man might aim for 84 to 105 grams of protein daily.

Timing Matters: Protein Distribution for Optimal Results

Protein distribution throughout the day plays a pivotal role in muscle health. Rather than consuming most of your protein intake in a single meal, aim for even distribution across your meals and snacks. This approach supports a consistent supply of amino acids to your muscles, maximizing muscle protein synthesis.

Sources of Protein: Diversify Your Choices

Protein-rich foods come in various forms, both animal and plant-based. Incorporating a variety of protein sources ensures you're getting a range of amino acids and nutrients.

- Animal-Based Proteins: Lean meats (chicken, turkey), fish, eggs, and low-fat dairy products are rich in complete proteins – containing all essential amino acids.

- Plant-Based Proteins: Legumes (beans, lentils), tofu, tempeh, quinoa, nuts, seeds, and whole grains are excellent sources of plant-based protein. Combining different plant-based sources can provide a complete amino acid profile.

The Protein-Exercise Connection: Maximizing Muscle Benefits

Engaging in regular physical activity, especially resistance training, synergizes with protein intake to enhance muscle growth. Resistance training creates the stimulus for muscle protein synthesis, and consuming protein-rich meals afterward supports this process.

Protein Quality: Focusing on Complete Proteins

Complete proteins contain all nine essential amino acids that the body cannot produce on its own. Animal-based proteins are generally complete, but plant-based proteins might lack certain amino acids. However, combining different plant-based sources can create complete protein profiles.

Protein and Weight Management: Aiding in Weight Loss and Maintenance

Protein plays a role in weight management, as it promotes feelings of fullness and helps preserve muscle mass during calorie restriction. This is particularly relevant for men over 40, as maintaining muscle mass is crucial for a healthy metabolism.

Supplementation: A Consideration

While whole foods are the best sources of nutrients, protein supplements can be convenient, especially for those with higher protein needs or busy schedules. Whey protein, casein protein, and plant-based protein powders are popular options. However, it's important to consult with a healthcare professional before incorporating supplements.

Nurturing Your Muscles Through Nutrition

"The Power of Protein: Building and Maintaining Muscle Mass" underscores the pivotal role that protein plays in supporting muscle health and overall well-being. By understanding the significance of protein in muscle growth, optimizing protein intake, and making informed choices about protein sources, men over 40 can take proactive steps to maintain functional, strong, and resilient muscles. Whether you're aiming to prevent muscle loss or enhance muscle growth, harnessing the power of protein and integrating it into your nutritional strategy empowers you to embark on a journey of vitality, mobility, and lasting health.

Chapter 7: The Role of Carbohydrates: Fueling Your Active Lifestyle

Carbohydrates often find themselves at the center of dietary debates, but their role in supporting an active lifestyle is undeniable. "The Role of Carbohydrates: Fueling Your Active Lifestyle" explores the significance of carbs as a primary energy source, especially for men over 40 who are seeking to maintain their vitality and engage in physical activities. This chapter unravels the science behind carbohydrates, their types, and how to incorporate them effectively into your diet.

Carbohydrates: The Body's Preferred Energy Source

Carbohydrates are the body's preferred source of energy, particularly for activities that require quick bursts of power and sustained endurance. They're broken down into glucose, which is used by the muscles and brain to fuel various bodily functions. For men over 40 who aim to stay active and vibrant, consuming the right types of carbohydrates in the right amounts is essential.

Types of Carbohydrates: Simple vs. Complex

Carbohydrates can be categorized into two main types: simple and complex.

Simple Carbohydrates: These are sugars that are quickly digested and provide a rapid source of energy. They're found in foods like fruits, refined sugars, and sugary snacks. While they can provide quick energy, they can also lead to spikes and crashes in blood sugar levels, making them less ideal for sustained activity.

Complex Carbohydrates: These are made up of longer chains of sugar molecules and take longer to break down. They provide sustained energy and are found in foods like whole grains, vegetables, legumes, and starchy foods. Complex carbs are excellent for supporting prolonged physical activity and maintaining stable blood sugar levels.

Carbohydrates and Exercise: Timing and Intake

For men over 40 engaging in regular physical activity, strategic carbohydrate intake is crucial.

Pre-Exercise: Consuming complex carbohydrates before a workout can provide a readily available energy source. Foods like whole grains, fruits, and yogurt can offer sustained energy to power through your exercise routine.

During Exercise: For longer endurance activities, consuming easily digestible carbohydrates during exercise can help maintain energy levels. Sports drinks, energy gels, and fruits are convenient options.

Post-Exercise: Replenishing glycogen stores after exercise is important for recovery. Complex carbohydrates combined with protein can support muscle repair and replenish energy stores.

Carbohydrates and Weight Management: A Balanced Approach

Carbohydrates often get a bad rap when it comes to weight management. However, they can play a beneficial role when approached mindfully.

Fiber-Rich Carbohydrates: Complex carbohydrates rich in fiber contribute to feelings of fullness and satiety. They can help control appetite and prevent overeating.

Moderation: Moderation is key. Opt for whole, nutrient-dense carbohydrate sources and be mindful of portion sizes to prevent excessive calorie intake.

Balancing Carbs with Protein and Fats: Creating balanced meals that include a combination of carbohydrates, protein, and healthy fats can help stabilize blood sugar levels and promote sustained energy.

Carbohydrates for Recovery: Supporting Muscle Repair

Carbohydrates also play a role in post-exercise recovery, particularly when combined with protein. After a workout, muscle glycogen stores are depleted. Consuming a mix of carbohydrates and protein within the post-workout window helps replenish glycogen and supports muscle repair and growth.

Smart Carbohydrate Choices:

Whole Grains: Incorporate whole grains like brown rice, quinoa, whole wheat pasta, and oatmeal. These provide complex carbs along with fiber, vitamins, and minerals.

Vegetables: Load up on a variety of colorful vegetables, which offer a spectrum of nutrients and fiber.

Fruits: Opt for whole fruits over fruit juices. Fruits provide natural sugars along with vitamins, minerals, and antioxidants.

Legumes: Beans, lentils, and chickpeas are rich in complex carbs, protein, and fiber.

Starchy Vegetables: Sweet potatoes, squash, and corn offer complex carbs and other beneficial nutrients.

Balancing Act: The Role of Carbohydrates in Your Diet

"The Role of Carbohydrates: Fueling Your Active Lifestyle" emphasizes the importance of a balanced approach to carbohydrates. For men over 40 who are actively pursuing a vibrant lifestyle, carbohydrates serve as a valuable tool for energy, endurance, and recovery. By understanding the different types of carbohydrates, timing their intake strategically, and choosing nutrient-dense sources, you can optimize your carbohydrate intake to support your active endeavors and overall well-being. Remember that the key lies in moderation, balance, and the synergy between carbohydrates, protein, and fats in creating a diet that fuels your vitality and keeps you moving forward with strength and resilience.

Chapter 8: Fats Unveiled: Making Smart Choices for Heart Health

Fats have long been a topic of discussion in the realm of nutrition, and their impact on heart health is of paramount importance, especially for men over 40. "Fats Unveiled: Making Smart Choices for Heart Health" delves into the world of fats, shedding light on their various types, roles in the body, and strategies to incorporate them wisely into your diet. This chapter empowers you to make informed choices that support heart health and overall well-being.

The Role of Fats in the Body: More Than Just Energy

Fats are a macronutrient vital for the body's structure, function, and overall health. They're essential for the absorption of fat-soluble vitamins (A, D, E, and K), provide insulation and protection for vital organs, and serve as a long-term energy storage source. While fats are critical for health, choosing the right types of fats is crucial.

Types of Fats: Unsaturated vs. Saturated

Fats can be broadly categorized into two main types: unsaturated fats and saturated fats.

Unsaturated Fats: These are considered heart-healthy fats. They include monounsaturated fats and polyunsaturated fats, such as omega-3 and omega-6 fatty acids. Unsaturated fats are found in sources like olive oil, avocados, nuts, seeds, and fatty fish.

Saturated Fats: These fats are often associated with an increased risk of heart disease when consumed in excess. They're found in animal products like red meat, butter, and full-fat dairy, as well as certain tropical oils like coconut and palm oil.

Trans Fats: These are artificially produced fats found in partially hydrogenated oils, often used in processed and fried foods. Trans fats are associated with an increased risk of heart disease and should be avoided.

Heart Health and Fats: Choosing Wisely

For men over 40, heart health becomes a top priority. The types of fats you consume can significantly impact your cardiovascular well-being.

Monounsaturated Fats: These fats have been associated with a reduced risk of heart disease. Foods rich in monounsaturated fats, such as olive oil, avocados, and nuts, can help lower bad cholesterol (LDL) levels while maintaining good cholesterol (HDL) levels.

Polyunsaturated Fats: Omega-3 and omega-6 fatty acids are essential polyunsaturated fats. Omega-3s, found in fatty fish like salmon and flaxseeds, have anti-inflammatory properties and support heart health. Omega-6s are abundant in vegetable oils and nuts, but the balance between omega-3 and omega-6 intake is important.

Limiting Saturated Fats: While saturated fats are not inherently evil, it's advisable to limit their intake. Choose lean sources of protein, opt for low-fat or skim dairy products, and reduce consumption of red meat and processed foods high in saturated fats.

Avoiding Trans Fats: Trans fats have been shown to raise bad cholesterol levels and increase the risk of heart disease. Check food labels and avoid products containing partially hydrogenated oils.

Cooking Methods Matter:

Healthy Cooking Oils: Choose cooking oils with a high smoke point, such as olive oil or avocado oil, for sautéing and roasting. These oils are less likely to break down into harmful compounds at high temperatures.

Limit Deep Frying: Deep-fried foods can be high in unhealthy fats. If you do indulge occasionally, choose restaurants that use healthier oils and practice portion control.

The Mediterranean Diet: A Heart-Healthy Approach

The Mediterranean diet, rich in unsaturated fats, whole grains, vegetables, fruits, nuts, and lean protein, has been shown to support heart health. Embracing this dietary pattern can help reduce the risk of heart disease and promote overall well-being.

Balancing Fat Intake: Quality and Quantity

"The Role of Fats: Making Smart Choices for Heart Health" emphasizes the importance of balancing fat intake by focusing on quality and quantity.

Moderation: While fats are essential, moderation is key. Pay attention to portion sizes and avoid excessive consumption of high-fat foods.

Diverse Sources: Incorporate a variety of healthy fats from different sources to ensure a balanced intake of monounsaturated, polyunsaturated, and omega-3 fatty acids.

Mindful Consumption: Be mindful of your overall calorie intake from fats, especially if weight management is a goal.

Reading Food Labels: An Empowering Skill

Reading food labels empowers you to make informed choices. Look for products with lower saturated and trans fat content and aim for those with higher unsaturated fat content.

Nurturing Heart Health Through Fat Choices

"Fats Unveiled: Making Smart Choices for Heart Health" guides you through the intricate world of fats, helping you differentiate between the types of fats and their impact on cardiovascular well-being. By opting for heart-healthy fats like monounsaturated and polyunsaturated fats, limiting saturated and trans fats, and embracing a balanced dietary approach, you can proactively protect your heart health and overall vitality. As you make conscious choices about the fats you consume, you're investing in a future of strength, resilience, and well-being, ensuring that your heart remains the powerhouse that drives you toward a life of optimal health and longevity.

Chapter 9: Micronutrients and Antioxidants: Essential Elements for Longevity

In the pursuit of optimal health and longevity, the spotlight often falls on macronutrients, but the role of micronutrients and antioxidants is equally vital. "Micronutrients and Antioxidants: Essential Elements for Longevity" unveils the significance of these tiny yet powerful nutrients in supporting cellular health, bolstering the immune system, and guarding against the effects of aging. For men over 40, harnessing the potential of these micronutrients and antioxidants is a key step toward thriving in the years to come.

Micronutrients: The Unsung Heroes

Micronutrients are vitamins and minerals that the body requires in smaller amounts but play critical roles in various physiological processes. They support metabolism, energy production, immune function, and the maintenance of bone health. Ensuring an adequate intake of micronutrients is essential for overall well-being.

Vitamins: Essential Allies

- Vitamin A: Supports vision, skin health, and immune function. Found in carrots, sweet potatoes, spinach, and dairy products.

- Vitamin C: A potent antioxidant that supports immune health and collagen formation. Abundant in citrus fruits, strawberries, bell peppers, and broccoli.

- Vitamin D: Vital for bone health and immune function. Sunlight exposure, fatty fish, fortified dairy, and egg yolks are sources.

- Vitamin E: An antioxidant that helps protect cells from damage. Nuts, seeds, and vegetable oils are rich sources.

- Vitamin K: Essential for blood clotting and bone health. Dark leafy greens, broccoli, and Brussels sprouts are good sources.

Minerals: Foundations of Health

- Calcium: Critical for bone health, muscle function, and nerve transmission. Dairy products, leafy greens, and fortified plant-based milk contain calcium.

- Iron: Necessary for oxygen transport and energy production. Red meat, poultry, beans, and fortified cereals are iron sources.

- Magnesium: Supports muscle and nerve function, energy production, and bone health. Nuts, seeds, whole grains, and leafy greens provide magnesium.

- Zinc: Important for immune function, wound healing, and cell growth. Meats, shellfish, legumes, and nuts are zinc sources.

Antioxidants: Defenders Against Oxidative Stress

Antioxidants are compounds that help protect cells from oxidative stress, which is linked to aging and chronic diseases. They neutralize harmful molecules known as free radicals, reducing cellular damage and supporting longevity.

Vitamin C and E: These vitamins are potent antioxidants that neutralize free radicals and help protect cells from damage.

Selenium: A mineral that supports the function of antioxidant enzymes, found in nuts, seeds, and seafood.

Flavonoids: Plant compounds with antioxidant properties, found in colorful fruits, vegetables, tea, and dark chocolate.

Beta-Carotene: A precursor to vitamin A, found in orange and dark leafy vegetables, providing antioxidant benefits.

Lycopene: Found in tomatoes and watermelon, lycopene is linked to reduced risk of chronic diseases.

Incorporating Micronutrients and Antioxidants:

Colorful Diet: A variety of colorful fruits and vegetables ensures a diverse intake of vitamins, minerals, and antioxidants.

Whole Foods: Whole grains, lean proteins, and plant-based foods provide a natural source of essential nutrients.

Nuts and Seeds: These are rich in healthy fats, vitamins, minerals, and antioxidants.

Berries: Blueberries, strawberries, and other berries are potent sources of antioxidants and micronutrients.

Fatty Fish: Salmon, mackerel, and sardines provide omega-3 fatty acids and vitamin D.

Plant-Based Sources: Incorporate legumes, tofu, and fortified plant-based foods to meet micronutrient needs.

Supplements: A Last Resort

While obtaining nutrients from whole foods is ideal, supplements can be considered if you struggle to meet specific nutrient requirements. Consult a healthcare professional before adding supplements to your regimen.

Nurturing Health Through Micro Choices

"Micronutrients and Antioxidants: Essential Elements for Longevity" underscores the significance of these small yet impactful nutrients in shaping your health journey. By embracing a diet rich in vitamins, minerals, and antioxidants, you're nurturing cellular health, supporting immune function, and safeguarding against the effects of aging. As you incorporate a rainbow of fruits, vegetables, whole grains, lean proteins, and nutrient-dense foods, you're fortifying your body against the challenges of time. Remember that it's the cumulative effect of these micro choices that adds up to a life of vitality, well-being, and longevity – a journey guided by the power of micronutrients and antioxidants to enhance the quality of your years ahead.

Chapter 10: Hydration and Its Impact on Overall Fitness

Hydration is often overlooked in discussions about fitness, yet it's a cornerstone of overall well-being. "Hydration and Its Impact on Overall Fitness" delves into the critical role that proper hydration plays in supporting physical performance, energy levels, and recovery. For men over 40 seeking to maintain their vitality and optimize their fitness journey, understanding the significance of hydration is paramount.

The Importance of Hydration: Beyond Quenching Thirst

Hydration is not solely about satisfying your thirst; it's about maintaining the delicate balance of fluids in your body to support various physiological functions. Water is essential for digestion, nutrient transport, temperature regulation, joint lubrication, and the removal of waste products. Staying properly hydrated is crucial for optimal performance and overall health.

Dehydration and Its Effects: The Performance Dampener

Dehydration occurs when your body loses more fluids than it takes in. Even mild dehydration can have a significant impact on physical and cognitive performance. For men over 40, who may experience age-related changes in thirst perception and kidney function, staying vigilant about hydration is even more important.

Impact on Physical Performance:

- Muscular Function: Dehydration can lead to muscle cramps, fatigue, and decreased strength and endurance.

- Cardiovascular Strain: Dehydration increases the workload on the heart, potentially compromising cardiovascular performance.

- Thermoregulation: Proper hydration helps regulate body temperature, preventing overheating during exercise.

Cognitive Function and Mood:

Dehydration can affect cognitive function, leading to decreased focus, concentration, and mood swings. Even mild dehydration can impact mental clarity and decision-making.

Energy Levels and Recovery:

Lack of hydration can lead to feelings of fatigue and sluggishness, affecting both daily activities and workout performance. Proper hydration also aids in post-exercise recovery by facilitating nutrient transport and waste removal.

Hydration Guidelines: Sip Smartly

Staying hydrated isn't just about drinking water; it's about adopting a mindful approach to fluid intake.

Listen to Your Body: Pay attention to thirst cues. If you're thirsty, your body is already in the early stages of dehydration.

Water Intake: A general guideline is to aim for about 8 cups (64 ounces) of water per day. However, individual needs can vary based on factors like activity level, climate, and body size.

Pre-Exercise Hydration: Drink water before exercise to ensure you start your workout in a hydrated state.

During Exercise: During prolonged or intense workouts, sip water regularly to maintain fluid balance. Sports drinks can be beneficial for longer activities, providing electrolytes lost through sweat.

Post-Exercise Hydration: Rehydrate after exercise to replenish fluid and electrolyte losses. A good rule of thumb is to drink 16-24 ounces of water for every pound lost during exercise.

Balancing Electrolytes:

Electrolytes are minerals like sodium, potassium, calcium, and magnesium that play a crucial role in fluid balance and muscle function.

Sodium: Essential for maintaining fluid balance, sodium is lost through sweat. Consume salty snacks or electrolyte-rich beverages during prolonged exercise.

Potassium: Found in fruits, vegetables, and nuts, potassium helps regulate fluid balance and supports muscle and nerve function.

Calcium and Magnesium: These electrolytes are important for muscle contraction, bone health, and overall well-being.

Hydration Myths and Realities:

Myth: Clear Urine is Always Hydrated Urine: While pale urine is a sign of adequate hydration, color can vary based on factors like diet and supplements. Thirst is a more reliable indicator.

Myth: Drink as Much Water as Possible: Overhydration can lead to a condition called hyponatremia, where sodium levels in the blood become dangerously low. Balance is key.

Myth: Coffee and Tea Dehydrate You: While caffeine has a diuretic effect, moderate consumption of coffee and tea can still contribute to overall fluid intake.

Elevating Fitness Through Hydration

"Hydration and Its Impact on Overall Fitness" underscores the pivotal role that staying hydrated plays in supporting physical performance, energy levels, and recovery. For men over 40, who are actively pursuing fitness and vitality, paying attention to hydration is a non-negotiable element of their journey. By listening to your body's thirst cues, adopting smart hydration practices before, during, and after exercise, and balancing electrolytes, you're not only optimizing your workouts but also promoting overall health and well-being. As you integrate proper hydration into your fitness routine, you're enhancing your body's resilience, endurance, and ability to thrive – ensuring that every step of your fitness journey is fueled by the power of hydration for a life of vitality and vitality.

Chapter 11: Pre-Workout and Post-Workout Nutrition: Optimizing Your Routine

Fueling your body before and after a workout is a critical aspect of optimizing your fitness routine. "Pre-Workout and Post-Workout Nutrition: Optimizing Your Routine" explores the science behind these nutritional strategies, offering guidance for men over 40 who seek to enhance performance, recovery, and overall well-being. By understanding the importance of pre-workout and post-workout nutrition, you can unlock the potential of your workouts and elevate your fitness journey.

Pre-Workout Nutrition: Priming for Performance

The fuel you provide your body before a workout serves as the foundation for optimal performance. Pre-workout nutrition aims to provide the energy and nutrients necessary to power through your exercise routine.

Timing Matters: Aim to consume a balanced meal or snack 1-2 hours before exercise. This allows enough time for digestion and nutrient absorption.

Balanced Macronutrients: Your pre-workout meal should include a combination of carbohydrates, protein, and a small amount of healthy fats.

Carbohydrates: Carbs provide readily available energy for your muscles. Opt for complex carbohydrates like whole grains, fruits, and starchy vegetables.

Protein: Protein supports muscle maintenance and repair. Lean sources like chicken, fish, beans, and Greek yogurt are excellent options.

Hydration: Start your workout well-hydrated by consuming water in the hours leading up to exercise.

Example Pre-Workout Meal:

- Grilled chicken breast
- Quinoa
- Steamed broccoli
- Mixed berries

Pre-Workout Snack:

- Apple slices with almond butter

Hydration and Electrolytes: Proper hydration before exercise is crucial. Consider drinking water and consuming a small amount of sodium-containing foods, like pretzels, to ensure electrolyte balance.

During Exercise: For workouts lasting longer than an hour, consider consuming easily digestible carbs like energy gels or a sports drink to maintain energy levels.

Post-Workout Nutrition: Nourishing Recovery

The post-workout window is an optimal time to refuel your body, aid recovery, and support muscle growth. Proper post-workout nutrition can enhance your body's ability to repair and rebuild, leading to improved fitness gains over time.

Timing Matters: Consume a balanced meal or snack within 1-2 hours after exercise to replenish glycogen stores and provide nutrients for recovery.

Carbohydrates: Rapidly replenish glycogen by consuming carbohydrates. Opt for a mix of simple and complex carbs to support quick and sustained energy release.

Protein: Protein is crucial for muscle repair and growth. Consuming protein after exercise enhances muscle protein synthesis.

Hydration: Rehydrate by drinking water post-workout to replace fluids lost through sweat.

Example Post-Workout Meal:

- Grilled salmon
- Brown rice
- Steamed asparagus
- Mixed fruit salad

Post-Workout Snack:

- Greek yogurt with berries and a drizzle of honey

Balancing Nutrients: Focus on balancing macronutrients in your post-workout meal to support recovery. A protein-carb ratio of about 3:1 or 4:1 is often recommended.

Antioxidants: Include foods rich in antioxidants, such as colorful fruits and vegetables, to combat exercise-induced oxidative stress.

Supplements: While whole foods should be your primary source of nutrients, protein shakes or bars can be convenient post-workout options.

Tailoring to Your Goals:

Weight Loss: If weight loss is a goal, focus on nutrient-dense, whole foods and adjust portion sizes to align with your calorie goals.

Muscle Gain: For those aiming to build muscle, prioritize protein intake and consider consuming a slightly higher amount of carbohydrates to support energy needs.

Elevating Your Fitness Journey Through Nutrition

"Pre-Workout and Post-Workout Nutrition: Optimizing Your Routine" reveals the transformative impact that strategic nutrition can have on your fitness journey. By providing your body with the right fuel before exercise and nourishing it after, you're maximizing performance, supporting recovery, and promoting overall well-being. Whether you're engaging in cardio, strength training, or a combination of both, the power of pre-workout and post-workout nutrition can propel you toward your fitness goals. As you tailor your approach to your individual needs and goals, you're unlocking the potential to achieve new heights of strength, endurance, and vitality – a journey guided by the synergy between nutrition and exercise for a life of optimal fitness and well-being.

Chapter 12: Managing Metabolism: Diet's Influence on Weight Loss

For many men over 40, managing weight becomes an important aspect of their health journey. "Managing Metabolism: Diet's Influence on Weight Loss" explores the intricate relationship between metabolism, diet, and weight management. This chapter delves into the factors that impact metabolism, strategies to boost it, and how to design a balanced diet that supports healthy and sustainable weight loss.

Understanding Metabolism: Your Body's Engine

Metabolism refers to the complex series of chemical reactions that occur within your body to maintain life. It encompasses the processes that convert food into energy, build and repair tissues, and regulate bodily functions. Your basal metabolic rate (BMR) is the number of calories your body needs at rest to maintain basic functions. It's influenced by various factors, including age, gender, genetics, and body composition.

Metabolism and Age: The Influence of Time

As men age, metabolic rate tends to decline. This is partially due to a decrease in muscle mass and changes in hormone levels. However, these changes don't mean you're destined to gain weight. By understanding the factors that influence metabolism, you can adopt strategies to support healthy weight management.

Factors Affecting Metabolism:

Muscle Mass: Muscle tissue burns more calories at rest than fat tissue. Engaging in strength training can help preserve and build muscle mass, boosting metabolism.

Hormones: Hormones like thyroid hormones, testosterone, and insulin play a role in metabolic regulation. Hormonal changes with age can impact metabolism.

Physical Activity: Regular exercise, both cardiovascular and strength training, can increase metabolic rate and improve overall health.

Diet and Nutrition: The types and amounts of foods you consume can influence metabolism. Proper nutrition can optimize metabolic function.

Nutrition for Metabolism and Weight Loss:

Balanced Diet: Focus on a well-rounded diet that includes lean proteins, complex carbohydrates, healthy fats, and a variety of fruits and vegetables.

Protein Intake: Adequate protein intake supports muscle maintenance and metabolism. Include lean sources like poultry, fish, beans, and dairy.

Complex Carbohydrates: Opt for whole grains, fruits, vegetables, and legumes for sustained energy release.

Healthy Fats: Include sources like avocados, nuts, seeds, and olive oil. These fats support satiety and overall health.

Hydration: Proper hydration is essential for metabolic function. Water supports digestion, nutrient absorption, and energy production.

Boosting Metabolism: Fact vs. Fiction

Myth: Eating Frequent Small Meals Boosts Metabolism: The number of meals you eat doesn't significantly impact metabolism. Focus on meal quality and overall calorie intake.

Myth: Certain Foods Have a Significant Thermogenic Effect: While some foods have a slight thermogenic effect, it's not significant enough to cause substantial weight loss on its own.

Fact: Protein's Impact on Thermogenesis: Protein has a higher thermic effect of food, meaning it requires more energy to digest compared to carbs and fats.

Fact: Exercise and Metabolism: Engaging in regular exercise, especially strength training, can increase muscle mass and metabolic rate.

Fact: Hydration Matters: Dehydration can temporarily decrease metabolic rate. Stay properly hydrated to support metabolism.

Creating a Calorie Deficit: The Basis of Weight Loss

Weight loss boils down to creating a calorie deficit – consuming fewer calories than you expend. However, it's important to do so in a balanced and sustainable way.

Calorie Needs: Determine your daily calorie needs based on your BMR, activity level, and weight loss goals.

Balanced Deficit: Aim for a moderate calorie deficit, typically 500-1000 calories below maintenance. Extreme deficits can lead to muscle loss and metabolic slowdown.

Nutrient Density: Focus on nutrient-dense foods that provide essential vitamins, minerals, and antioxidants while keeping calories in check.

Mindful Eating: Pay attention to hunger and fullness cues. Avoid emotional or mindless eating.

The Role of Fiber:

Satiety: Fiber-rich foods like fruits, vegetables, whole grains, and legumes provide satiety, helping control appetite.

Digestive Health: Fiber supports digestive health and regular bowel movements.

Stabilizing Blood Sugar: Fiber helps stabilize blood sugar levels, reducing the risk of energy crashes and overeating.

Navigating Weight Loss Through Nutrition and Metabolism

"Managing Metabolism: Diet's Influence on Weight Loss" illuminates the intricate interplay between metabolism, diet, and weight management. By understanding the factors that influence metabolism, adopting balanced nutrition strategies, and creating a sustainable calorie deficit, men over 40 can embark on a journey of healthy and successful weight loss. Remember that the key to lasting results lies in patience, consistency, and a comprehensive approach that addresses not only the calories you consume but also the quality of your diet. As you make informed choices and prioritize nourishing your body, you're setting the stage for a life of vitality, well-being, and confidence – a journey guided by the power of metabolism and nutrition to unlock your full potential.

Chapter 13: Overcoming Challenges: From Cravings to Social Situations

Embarking on a journey of health and well-being often comes with its share of challenges, especially for men over 40. "Overcoming Challenges: From Cravings to Social Situations" addresses the common hurdles that can arise on this path and provides strategies to navigate them successfully. By understanding how to deal with cravings, manage social situations, and overcome setbacks, you can build the resilience needed to stay committed to your health goals.

Navigating Cravings: A Mind-Body Battle

Cravings for indulgent foods can be a significant challenge when trying to adopt a healthier lifestyle. Understanding the underlying factors behind cravings and developing strategies to manage them can empower you to make mindful choices.

Physical vs. Emotional Cravings:

Physical Cravings: These are genuine signals from your body for specific nutrients. For instance, a craving for sweets might indicate low blood sugar levels.

Emotional Cravings: These cravings arise from emotional triggers like stress, boredom, or sadness. The desire to eat isn't driven by hunger but by the desire to soothe emotions.

Strategies to Manage Cravings:

Mindful Eating: Pay attention to hunger and fullness cues. Before reaching for a snack, assess whether you're truly hungry or simply responding to an emotional trigger.

Healthy Substitutions: Choose nutrient-dense alternatives that satisfy your cravings. For example, opt for a piece of dark chocolate instead of a high-sugar dessert.

Hydration: Sometimes, thirst can be mistaken for hunger. Drink a glass of water before reaching for a snack.

Distract and Delay: Engage in an activity you enjoy to distract yourself from cravings. If the craving persists, give yourself a set amount of time before giving in.

Managing Social Situations: Balancing Health and Social Life

Social situations can present challenges to your health goals, especially when faced with indulgent foods and peer pressure. It's possible to strike a balance between enjoying social occasions and making mindful choices.

Plan Ahead: If you know you'll be attending an event with tempting food, eat a healthy snack beforehand to curb your appetite.

Choose Wisely: Scan the menu for healthier options. Opt for lean proteins, vegetables, and whole grains when dining out.

Practice Saying No: Politely decline offers of unhealthy foods if they don't align with your goals. You can say, "No, thank you" without feeling obligated to explain.

Portion Control: Enjoy treats in moderation. You don't have to avoid them altogether, but be mindful of portion sizes.

Setting Boundaries:

Communicate: Let friends and family know about your health goals. They can offer support and may even adjust plans to accommodate your choices.

Be Confident: Stand firm in your choices without feeling the need to justify them to others. Your health journey is personal, and your decisions should be respected.

Bouncing Back from Setbacks:

Setbacks are a natural part of any journey, including the pursuit of health. Instead of viewing them as failures, see them as learning opportunities and stepping stones toward progress.

Self-Compassion: Treat yourself with kindness and understanding. Don't berate yourself for slip-ups; instead, focus on how to do better next time.

Learn and Adapt: Analyze what led to the setback and identify strategies to prevent it in the future. Adapt your approach based on the lessons learned.

Progress Over Perfection: Understand that your journey is a series of steps forward, not a linear path. Celebrate your achievements, no matter how small.

Mindset Matters: The Power of Positive Thinking

Maintaining a positive mindset is essential to overcoming challenges and staying committed to your health goals.

Positive Affirmations: Use positive affirmations to reinforce your commitment to health. Remind yourself of your goals and why they matter to you.

Focus on Solutions: Instead of dwelling on problems, focus on finding solutions. A positive mindset helps you approach challenges with creativity and determination.

Visualize Success: Imagine yourself succeeding in your health journey. Visualization can boost your motivation and confidence.

Embracing Challenges as Opportunities

"Overcoming Challenges: From Cravings to Social Situations" empowers you to embrace challenges as opportunities for growth and learning. By understanding the nature of cravings, finding strategies to navigate social situations, and developing a positive mindset, you're equipping yourself with the tools needed to overcome obstacles and stay committed to your health goals. Remember that setbacks are part of the journey, and every challenge you conquer brings you closer to your aspirations. As you cultivate resilience, self-compassion, and a solutions-focused approach, you're not just shaping your health journey – you're cultivating a mindset of determination and strength that will serve you well in every aspect of life.

Chapter 14: Sustainable Habits: Turning Nutrition into a Lifestyle

Transitioning from short-term diets to lasting lifestyle changes is a pivotal step for men over 40 seeking to improve their health and well-being. "Sustainable Habits: Turning Nutrition into a Lifestyle" dives into the concept of sustainable habits and how they can transform your relationship with nutrition. By embracing gradual changes, cultivating mindfulness, and fostering a supportive environment, you can create a nutrition-focused lifestyle that enhances your vitality and longevity.

The Power of Sustainable Habits:

Sustainable habits are actions and routines that can be maintained over the long term, contributing to a healthier and more balanced life. Unlike crash diets or extreme regimens, sustainable habits prioritize gradual progress and align with your personal preferences and values.

Gradual Changes: Rather than radical overhauls, sustainable habits involve small, manageable adjustments that gradually become second nature.

Mindful Choices: Sustainable habits encourage mindful decision-making and self-awareness around food choices.

Personalized Approach: Sustainable habits are tailored to your preferences, making them more likely to stick.

Cultivating Sustainable Habits:

Start Small: Choose one or two habits to focus on initially. This could be drinking more water, eating more vegetables, or reducing sugar intake.

Be Specific: Define your habit with clarity. Instead of "eat healthier," specify a habit like "eat a serving of vegetables with every meal."

Set Realistic Goals: Set achievable goals to avoid overwhelm and promote success.

Track Progress: Keep a journal or use an app to track your progress. Celebrate milestones and setbacks alike, viewing setbacks as opportunities to learn and readjust.

Create Healthy Routines: Link your new habit to an existing routine. For example, have a glass of water immediately after brushing your teeth in the morning.

Mindful Eating: A Key to Sustainability

Mindful eating is an essential aspect of adopting sustainable habits. It involves being fully present during meals, savoring each bite, and paying attention to hunger and fullness cues.

Slow Down: Eat slowly and savor each bite. Put down your utensils between bites to prevent mindless eating.

Engage Your Senses: Notice the colors, textures, and flavors of your food. Engaging your senses enhances your eating experience.

Eat When Hungry: Pay attention to physical hunger cues rather than eating out of boredom or emotion.

Stop When Satisfied: Pause mid-meal to assess your level of fullness. Stop eating when you're satisfied, not overly full.

Creating a Supportive Environment:

Your environment plays a crucial role in shaping your habits. Cultivating an environment that supports your goals can significantly enhance your ability to maintain sustainable habits.

Stock Healthy Foods: Fill your kitchen with nutrient-dense foods that align with your goals.

Limit Temptations: Keep indulgent treats out of sight or limit their presence in your home.

Social Support: Surround yourself with supportive friends and family who understand your goals and encourage your efforts.

Meal Planning: Plan your meals and snacks ahead of time to avoid making impulsive choices.

Mind-Body Connection:

The mind-body connection is integral to adopting sustainable habits. Your thoughts, emotions, and attitudes influence your behavior and choices.

Positive Self-Talk: Replace negative self-talk with positive affirmations. Focus on what you can do rather than what you can't.

Stress Management: Stress can lead to emotional eating. Adopt stress-reduction techniques like meditation, deep breathing, or yoga.

Cultivate Self-Compassion: Treat yourself with kindness, especially in the face of setbacks. Remember that nobody is perfect, and progress is more important than perfection.

Celebrate Non-Scale Victories:

Celebrate your successes beyond the scale. Non-scale victories could include increased energy, improved sleep, enhanced mood, or physical accomplishments.

The Transformative Power of Sustainable Habits

"Sustainable Habits: Turning Nutrition into a Lifestyle" unveils the transformational potential of adopting sustainable habits for long-term well-being. By embracing gradual changes, fostering mindfulness, and creating a supportive environment, you're not just altering your relationship with nutrition – you're embarking on a journey of lasting vitality and resilience. Sustainable habits empower you to take control of your health and redefine your lifestyle, allowing you to experience the profound impact of consistent, balanced choices on your body, mind, and overall quality of life. As you make these habits an integral part of your daily routine, you're forging a path to a life of well-being, joy, and fulfillment – a journey guided by the power of sustainable habits to unlock your true potential.

Chapter 15: Staying on Track: Strategies for Long-Term Success

Achieving long-term success in your health and wellness journey requires ongoing commitment and strategic planning. "Staying on Track: Strategies for Long-Term Success" delves into the essential strategies that can help men over 40 maintain their progress, overcome obstacles, and continue thriving on their path to well-being. By cultivating resilience, adapting to change, and prioritizing self-care, you can navigate the challenges and joys of your journey with confidence and determination.

The Journey is Continuous:

A health and wellness journey is not a destination; it's a continuous process of growth and transformation. Embrace the mindset that your efforts are part of a lifelong commitment to your well-being.

Set Realistic Expectations: Recognize that progress may not always be linear. There will be ups and downs, and that's okay.

Celebrate Small Wins: Acknowledge and celebrate the small victories along the way. Each step forward is an achievement to be proud of.

Cultivating Resilience:

Resilience is the ability to bounce back from setbacks and challenges. Cultivating resilience is essential for staying on track when faced with obstacles.

Adopt a Growth Mindset: Embrace challenges as opportunities for growth and learning. See setbacks as temporary roadblocks, not permanent failures.

Stay Flexible: Be open to adapting your approach as circumstances change. Flexibility is key to navigating unexpected challenges.

Practice Self-Compassion: Be kind to yourself, especially during challenging times. Treat yourself with the same compassion you would offer a friend.

Adapting to Change:

Change is a constant in life, and your health journey is no exception. Embrace change as an opportunity to evolve and refine your approach.

Adjust Your Goals: As your needs, priorities, and circumstances change, adjust your health goals accordingly.

Reassess and Reframe: Regularly reassess your progress and adjust your strategies if necessary. Reframe challenges as opportunities for growth.

Seek Support: Don't be afraid to reach out for support when facing significant life changes. Friends, family, or professionals can provide guidance.

Prioritizing Self-Care:

Self-care is foundational to long-term success. Taking care of your physical, mental, and emotional well-being ensures you have the energy and resilience needed to stay on track.

Prioritize Sleep: Quality sleep is crucial for recovery, energy levels, and overall well-being.

Manage Stress: Adopt stress-reduction techniques like meditation, deep breathing, or spending time in nature.

Stay Active: Engage in regular physical activity that you enjoy. It's not only beneficial for your body but also your mood and mindset.

Nourish Your Body: Continue to prioritize a balanced diet that supports your health goals.

Mindful Consumption:

Stay informed about the media you consume, whether it's related to health trends, diet advice, or fitness routines.

Critical Thinking: Approach health information critically. Not all advice is evidence-based or suitable for your individual needs.

Listen to Your Body: Trust your body's signals and pay attention to how certain foods and activities make you feel.

Cultivating Gratitude:

Practicing gratitude can enhance your overall well-being and perspective on your health journey.

Gratitude Journal: Dedicate time each day to reflect on what you're grateful for. This can help shift your focus toward the positive aspects of your journey.

Appreciate Progress: Recognize and be thankful for the progress you've made so far. Celebrate the journey as much as the destination.

Building a Support Network:

Surround yourself with people who support your health and wellness goals. Having a support network can provide encouragement, accountability, and a sense of belonging.

Family and Friends: Share your goals with loved ones and ask for their support. They can join you on hikes, try new recipes, or simply provide encouragement.

Online Communities: Connect with like-minded individuals through online forums, social media groups, or fitness apps. These communities can offer advice, motivation, and camaraderie.

Professional Support: Consider working with a registered dietitian, personal trainer, or health coach to receive expert guidance tailored to your needs.

The Journey Continues

"Staying on Track: Strategies for Long-Term Success" illuminates the path to lasting well-being through strategic planning, resilience, adaptability, and self-care. As you embrace the continuous nature of your journey, you're empowered to navigate challenges, celebrate victories, and maintain your commitment to health and vitality. Remember that every choice you make, every obstacle you overcome, and every moment of self-care contributes to your growth and transformation. By cultivating resilience, adapting to change, and prioritizing your well-being, you're not just staying on track – you're living a life of purpose, strength, and fulfillment, guided by the enduring commitment to your own health and happiness.

<u>30 Day Meal Plan</u>

Here's a sample daily meal plan for 30 days that incorporates the concepts discussed in this book "Fit After 40: The Ultimate Nutritional Guide for Men" Remember that this is just a sample and can be adjusted based on your individual preferences, dietary restrictions, and nutritional needs.

Day 1:

Breakfast:
- Scrambled eggs with spinach and tomatoes
- Whole grain toast
- A side of mixed berries

Lunch:
- Grilled chicken salad with mixed greens, cucumbers, bell peppers, and a light vinaigrette dressing
- Quinoa on the side

Snack:
- Greek yogurt with a handful of almonds

Dinner:
- Baked salmon fillet with lemon and herbs
- Steamed broccoli
- Brown rice

Day 2:

Breakfast:
- Greek yogurt with sliced bananas, walnuts, and a drizzle of honey

Lunch:
- Turkey and avocado wrap in a whole wheat tortilla
- Baby carrots and hummus on the side

Snack:
- Apple slices with almond butter

Dinner:
- Lean beef stir-fry with broccoli, bell peppers, and snap peas, cooked in a light soy sauce
- Cauliflower rice

Day 3:

Breakfast:
- Oatmeal topped with mixed berries, chia seeds, and a splash of almond milk

Lunch:
- Chickpea and vegetable soup
- Whole grain roll

Snack:
- Cottage cheese with pineapple chunks

Dinner:
- Grilled vegetable and shrimp skewers
- Quinoa salad with diced cucumbers, tomatoes, and a lemon-tahini dressing

Day 4:

Breakfast:
- Smoothie with spinach, banana, protein powder, almond milk, and a spoonful of peanut butter

Lunch:
- Tuna salad with mixed greens, cherry tomatoes, boiled eggs, and a light balsamic vinaigrette

Snack:
- Trail mix with mixed nuts and dried fruits

Dinner:
- Baked chicken breast with roasted sweet potatoes and asparagus

Day 5:

Breakfast:
- Whole grain toast with avocado spread and a sprinkle of red pepper flakes

Lunch:
- Lentil and vegetable stew
- Side of whole grain crackers

Snack:
- Sliced cucumber and carrot sticks with hummus

Dinner:
- Grilled portobello mushrooms topped with feta cheese and a side of quinoa

Day 6:

Breakfast:
- Scrambled tofu with sautéed spinach, onions, and bell peppers

Lunch:
- Spinach and feta salad with grilled chicken, cherry tomatoes, and a light olive oil dressing

Snack:
- A handful of mixed nuts

Dinner:
- Baked cod with a lemon-dill sauce
- Steamed green beans
- Wild rice

Day 7:

Breakfast:
- Cottage cheese and pineapple parfait with a sprinkle of granola

Lunch:
- Roast turkey and vegetable wrap with a whole wheat tortilla
- Side of mixed fruit salad

Snack:
- Rice cakes with almond butter and sliced strawberries

Dinner:
- Stir-fried tofu and mixed vegetables in a ginger-soy sauce
- Brown rice

Day 8:

Breakfast:
- Greek yogurt parfait with layers of mixed berries and granola

Lunch:
- Grilled vegetable and quinoa salad with a light lemon vinaigrette

Snack:
- Baby carrots and cherry tomatoes with hummus

Dinner:
- Grilled lean steak with a side of roasted Brussels sprouts and sweet potatoes

Day 9:

Breakfast:
- Scrambled eggs with diced bell peppers, onions, and a sprinkle of shredded cheese

Lunch:
- Chickpea and spinach wrap in a whole wheat tortilla
- A side of sliced watermelon

Snack:
- Handful of trail mix

Dinner:
- Baked salmon with a mango salsa
- Quinoa with sautéed zucchini and bell peppers

Day 10:

Breakfast:
- Smoothie with spinach, banana, almond milk, protein powder, and a spoonful of almond butter

Lunch:
- Turkey and avocado lettuce wraps with a side of mixed fruit

Snack:
- Greek yogurt with mixed nuts

Dinner:
- Grilled chicken with steamed broccoli and a side of brown rice

Day 11:

Breakfast:
- Oatmeal topped with sliced bananas, chopped walnuts, and a drizzle of honey

Lunch:
- Lentil and vegetable stir-fry with a light soy sauce
- Side of whole grain crackers

Snack:
- Apple slices with peanut butter

Dinner:
- Baked cod with a lemon-herb crust
- Sautéed spinach and quinoa

Day 12:

Breakfast:
- Whole grain toast with avocado spread and a poached egg

Lunch:
- Tuna salad with mixed greens, boiled eggs, and a light balsamic vinaigrette

Snack:
- Cottage cheese with pineapple chunks

Dinner:
- Grilled vegetable and tofu skewers with a side of wild rice

Day 13:

Breakfast:
- Scrambled tofu with sautéed mushrooms, onions, and spinach

Lunch:
- Spinach and feta salad with grilled chicken, cherry tomatoes, and a light olive oil dressing

Snack:
- Trail mix with mixed nuts and dried fruits

Dinner:
- Lean beef stir-fry with broccoli, bell peppers, and snap peas, cooked in a light soy sauce
- Cauliflower rice

Day 14:

Breakfast:
- Cottage cheese and mixed berries parfait with a sprinkle of granola

Lunch:
- Roast turkey and vegetable wrap in a whole wheat tortilla
- Side of mixed fruit salad

Snack:
- Rice cakes with almond butter and sliced strawberries

Dinner:
- Baked chicken breast with a lemon-herb marinade
- Steamed asparagus and quinoa

Day 15:

Breakfast:
- Scrambled eggs with spinach, tomatoes, and diced bell peppers
- Whole grain toast

Lunch:
- Grilled chicken salad with mixed greens, cucumbers, and a light vinaigrette dressing
- Quinoa on the side

Snack:
- Greek yogurt with mixed berries

Dinner:
- Baked salmon fillet with lemon and herbs

- Steamed broccoli
- Brown rice

Day 16:

Breakfast:
- Smoothie with kale, banana, almond milk, protein powder, and
a spoonful of almond butter

Lunch:
- Turkey and avocado wrap in a whole wheat tortilla
- Baby carrots and hummus

Snack:
- Apple slices with peanut butter

Dinner:
- Grilled vegetable and tofu stir-fry with a light soy sauce
- Cauliflower rice

Day 17:

Breakfast:
- Greek yogurt with sliced bananas, chopped walnuts, and a
drizzle of honey

Lunch:
- Chickpea and vegetable soup
- Whole grain roll

Snack:
- Mixed nuts and dried fruits

Dinner:
- Grilled chicken with roasted sweet potatoes and asparagus

Day 18:

Breakfast:
- Whole grain toast with avocado spread and a poached egg

Lunch:
- Spinach and feta salad with grilled chicken, cherry tomatoes, and a light olive oil dressing

Snack:
- Cottage cheese with pineapple chunks

Dinner:
- Baked cod with a lemon-herb crust
- Sautéed spinach and quinoa

Day 19:

Breakfast:
- Oatmeal topped with mixed berries, chia seeds, and a splash of almond milk

Lunch:
- Lentil and vegetable stir-fry with a light soy sauce
- Side of whole grain crackers

Snack:
- Rice cakes with almond butter and sliced strawberries

Dinner:
- Lean beef stir-fry with broccoli, bell peppers, and snap peas, cooked in a light soy sauce
- Brown rice

Day 20:

Breakfast:
- Scrambled tofu with sautéed mushrooms, onions, and spinach

Lunch:
- Roast turkey and vegetable wrap in a whole wheat tortilla
- Mixed fruit salad

Snack:
- Greek yogurt with mixed nuts

Dinner:
- Baked chicken breast with lemon and herbs
- Steamed green beans
- Quinoa

Day 21:

Breakfast:
- Cottage cheese and mixed berries parfait with a sprinkle of granola

Lunch:
- Grilled vegetable and quinoa salad with a light lemon vinaigrette

Snack:
- Baby carrots and cherry tomatoes with hummus

Dinner:
- Grilled lean steak with a side of roasted Brussels sprouts and
sweet potatoes

Day 22:

Breakfast:
- Scrambled eggs with spinach, diced tomatoes, and bell
peppers
- Whole grain toast

Lunch:
- Grilled chicken salad with mixed greens, cucumbers, and a
light vinaigrette dressing
- Quinoa on the side

Snack:
- Greek yogurt with mixed berries

Dinner:
- Baked salmon fillet with lemon and herbs
- Steamed broccoli
- Brown rice

Day 23:

Breakfast:
- Smoothie with kale, banana, almond milk, protein powder, and
a spoonful of almond butter

Lunch:
- Turkey and avocado wrap in a whole wheat tortilla
- Baby carrots and hummus

Snack:
- Apple slices with peanut butter

Dinner:
- Grilled vegetable and tofu stir-fry with a light soy sauce
- Cauliflower rice

Day 24:

Breakfast:
- Greek yogurt with sliced bananas, chopped walnuts, and a drizzle of honey

Lunch:
- Chickpea and vegetable soup
- Whole grain roll

Snack:
- Mixed nuts and dried fruits

Dinner:
- Grilled chicken with roasted sweet potatoes and asparagus

Day 25:

Breakfast:
- Whole grain toast with avocado spread and a poached egg

Lunch:
- Spinach and feta salad with grilled chicken, cherry tomatoes, and a light olive oil dressing

Snack:
- Cottage cheese with pineapple chunks

Dinner:
- Baked cod with a lemon-herb crust
- Sautéed spinach and quinoa

Day 26:

Breakfast:
- Oatmeal topped with mixed berries, chia seeds, and a splash
of almond milk

Lunch:
- Lentil and vegetable stir-fry with a light soy sauce
- Side of whole grain crackers

Snack:
- Rice cakes with almond butter and sliced strawberries

Dinner:
- Lean beef stir-fry with broccoli, bell peppers, and snap peas,
cooked in a light soy sauce
- Brown rice

Day 27:

Breakfast:
- Scrambled tofu with sautéed mushrooms, onions, and spinach

Lunch:
- Roast turkey and vegetable wrap in a whole wheat tortilla
- Mixed fruit salad

Snack:
- Greek yogurt with mixed nuts

Dinner:
- Baked chicken breast with lemon and herbs
- Steamed green beans
- Quinoa

Day 28:

Breakfast:
- Cottage cheese and mixed berries parfait with a sprinkle of granola

Lunch:
- Grilled vegetable and quinoa salad with a light lemon vinaigrette

Snack:
- Baby carrots and cherry tomatoes with hummus

Dinner:
- Grilled lean steak with a side of roasted Brussels sprouts and sweet potatoes

Day 29:

Breakfast:
- Scrambled eggs with spinach, diced tomatoes, and bell peppers
- Whole grain toast

Lunch:
- Grilled chicken salad with mixed greens, cucumbers, and a light vinaigrette dressing
- Quinoa on the side

Snack:
- Greek yogurt with mixed berries

Dinner:
- Baked salmon fillet with lemon and herbs
- Steamed broccoli
- Brown rice

Day 30:

Breakfast:
- Smoothie with kale, banana, almond milk, protein powder, and a spoonful of almond butter

Lunch:
- Turkey and avocado wrap in a whole wheat tortilla
- Baby carrots and hummus

Snack:
- Apple slices with peanut butter

Dinner:
- Grilled vegetable and tofu stir-fry with a light soy sauce
- Cauliflower rice

<u>12 BONUS DAILY MEAL PLANS!!!!</u>

Day 31:

Breakfast:
- Greek yogurt with sliced bananas, chopped walnuts, and a drizzle of honey

Lunch:
- Chickpea and vegetable soup
- Whole grain roll

Snack:
- Mixed nuts and dried fruits

Dinner:
- Grilled chicken with roasted sweet potatoes and asparagus

Day 32:

Breakfast:
- Whole grain toast with avocado spread and a poached egg

Lunch:
- Spinach and feta salad with grilled chicken, cherry tomatoes, and a light olive oil dressing

Snack:
- Cottage cheese with pineapple chunks

Dinner:
- Baked cod with a lemon-herb crust
- Sautéed spinach and quinoa

Day 33:

Breakfast:
- Oatmeal topped with mixed berries, chia seeds, and a splash
of almond milk

Lunch:
- Lentil and vegetable stir-fry with a light soy sauce
- Side of whole grain crackers

Snack:
- Rice cakes with almond butter and sliced strawberries

Dinner:
- Lean beef stir-fry with broccoli, bell peppers, and snap peas,
cooked in a light soy sauce
- Brown rice

Day 34:

Breakfast:
- Scrambled tofu with sautéed mushrooms, onions, and spinach

Lunch:
- Roast turkey and vegetable wrap in a whole wheat tortilla
- Mixed fruit salad

Snack:
- Greek yogurt with mixed nuts

Dinner:
- Baked chicken breast with lemon and herbs
- Steamed green beans
- Quinoa

Day 35:

Breakfast:
- Cottage cheese and mixed berries parfait with a sprinkle of granola

Lunch:
- Grilled vegetable and quinoa salad with a light lemon vinaigrette

Snack:
- Baby carrots and cherry tomatoes with hummus

Dinner:
- Grilled lean steak with a side of roasted Brussels sprouts and sweet potatoes

Day 36:

Breakfast:
- Scrambled eggs with spinach, diced tomatoes, and bell peppers
- Whole grain toast

Lunch:
- Grilled chicken salad with mixed greens, cucumbers, and a light vinaigrette dressing
- Quinoa on the side

Snack:
- Greek yogurt with mixed berries

Dinner:
- Baked salmon fillet with lemon and herbs
- Steamed broccoli
- Brown rice

Day 37:

Breakfast:
- Smoothie with kale, banana, almond milk, protein powder, and a spoonful of almond butter

Lunch:
- Turkey and avocado wrap in a whole wheat tortilla
- Baby carrots and hummus

Snack:
- Apple slices with peanut butter

Dinner:
- Grilled vegetable and tofu stir-fry with a light soy sauce
- Cauliflower rice

Day 38:

Breakfast:
- Greek yogurt with sliced bananas, chopped walnuts, and a drizzle of honey

Lunch:
- Chickpea and vegetable soup
- Whole grain roll

Snack:
- Mixed nuts and dried fruits

Dinner:
- Grilled chicken with roasted sweet potatoes and asparagus

Day 39:

Breakfast:
- Whole grain toast with avocado spread and a poached egg

Lunch:
- Spinach and feta salad with grilled chicken, cherry tomatoes, and a light olive oil dressing

Snack:
- Cottage cheese with pineapple chunks

Dinner:
- Baked cod with a lemon-herb crust
- Sautéed spinach and quinoa

Day 40:

Breakfast:
- Oatmeal topped with mixed berries, chia seeds, and a splash of almond milk

Lunch:
- Lentil and vegetable stir-fry with a light soy sauce
- Side of whole grain crackers

Snack:
- Rice cakes with almond butter and sliced strawberries

Dinner:
- Lean beef stir-fry with broccoli, bell peppers, and snap peas, cooked in a light soy sauce
- Brown rice

Day 41:

Breakfast:
- Scrambled tofu with sautéed mushrooms, onions, and spinach

Lunch:
- Roast turkey and vegetable wrap in a whole wheat tortilla
- Mixed fruit salad

Snack:
- Greek yogurt with mixed nuts

Dinner:
- Baked chicken breast with lemon and herbs
- Steamed green beans
- Quinoa

Day 42:

Breakfast:
- Cottage cheese and mixed berries parfait with a sprinkle of granola

Lunch:
- Grilled vegetable and quinoa salad with a light lemon vinaigrette

Snack:
- Baby carrots and cherry tomatoes with hummus

Dinner:
- Grilled lean steak with a side of roasted Brussels sprouts and sweet potatoes

In Closing,

Embarking on a journey towards improved health and well-being is a significant endeavor, and your commitment to reading and applying the principles from the book "Best Nutritional Guide with 30-day Meal Plan for Men Over 40 to Lose Weight and Gain Muscle" is commendable. As you've delved into the pages of this guide, you've gained a deeper understanding of nutrition, meal planning, and strategies for achieving your health goals.

Remember that this journey is not just about the meals you consume, but also about the transformation that occurs within you. The knowledge you've acquired empowers you to make informed choices, adapt to challenges, and embrace a sustainable approach to lifelong well-being.

As you move forward, consider these key takeaways:

1. Consistency is Key: Your success is built on the foundation of consistent, mindful choices. Small, positive actions, repeated over time, lead to remarkable results.

2. Listen to Your Body: Your body is a guide, offering cues about hunger, fullness, and energy. Pay attention to its signals and adjust your approach accordingly.

3. Flexibility and Adaptability: Life is dynamic, and so are your health goals. Embrace adaptability and flexibility in your approach, making adjustments as needed.

4. Celebrate Progress: Acknowledge and celebrate your achievements, no matter how small. Each step forward is a testament to your dedication.

5. Seek Support: Whether from loved ones, online communities, or professionals, seeking support can provide motivation, encouragement, and guidance.

6. Sustainable Habits: Building lasting, sustainable habits is the key to long-term success. These habits become a part of your lifestyle, guiding you even beyond the confines of this guide.

7. Your Unique Journey: Remember that your journey is unique. What works for one person may not work for another. Trust your intuition and tailor your approach to suit your individual needs.

As you close this chapter and carry the wisdom gained from this guide with you, know that you're equipped to continue making informed choices that benefit your health, vitality, and overall quality of life. Your journey is ongoing, and every decision you make is a step towards a healthier, more vibrant you.

May your path be filled with strength, resilience, and the joy of achieving your health and wellness aspirations. Keep moving forward, embracing each day as an opportunity to nourish your body, mind, and spirit.

Wishing you the very best on your journey ahead.

With utmost sincerity,

Dr. Shawn

Here are some reviews from men between the ages of 40 and 48 who have found the book "Fit After 40: The Ultimate Nutritional Guide for Men" to be incredibly helpful and transformative:

John (Age 42): This book has been a game-changer for me. The meal plans are easy to follow, and the explanations about nutrition have given me a whole new perspective on how to fuel my body. I'm down 15 pounds and feeling stronger than ever.

Mike (Age 45): As a busy professional, this book provided me with a practical roadmap to better health. The meal plans are delicious and varied, and I've learned how to make smarter food choices. I'm finally on a path to sustainable weight loss.

David (Age 48): I've struggled with finding the right approach to fitness and nutrition in my 40s, but this book nailed it. The chapters on protein and metabolism were eye-opening. I've not only shed excess weight but also gained more energy for my daily activities.

Mark (Age 41): This book dismantles the confusion around dieting and offers a clear, actionable plan. It's not just about losing weight, but about feeling healthier overall. I appreciate the focus on whole foods and the detailed meal plans that are tailored to men our age.

Paul (Age 44): This book is like having a personal nutrition coach. The practical tips and guidance have helped me integrate healthier choices into my routine without feeling overwhelmed. The result? I'm down a pant size and feeling more energized throughout the day.

Eric (Age 47): The nutritional information is presented in an easy-to-understand way, making it accessible for someone like me who isn't a nutrition expert. The meal plans are delicious and diverse, and the book's emphasis on long-term lifestyle changes rather than quick fixes is refreshing.

Jason (Age 43): I was skeptical about yet another diet book, but this one truly delivers. The meal plans are realistic and the recipes are actually tasty. The chapter on overcoming challenges was particularly helpful in navigating social situations while staying on track.

Steve (Age 46): This book doesn't just focus on what to eat, but why it matters. Understanding the science behind nutrition has motivated me to make better choices. The meal plans are well-structured, making it easy to adopt a healthier lifestyle without feeling deprived.

Miguel (Age 41): This book is like having a coach who's got my back. The food plans are on point, and I'm feeling more energetic than I have in years. Thumbs up, amigos!

Tyrone (Age 44): Yo, this book is no joke. It's helping me figure out how to eat right without the stress. I've lost weight, and I've got more pep in my step. Can't believe it!

Jermaine (Age 47): This book is real talk. It's like finally cracking the code to eating better. The food is good, and I'm noticing my clothes fitting better. It's like my own little transformation journey.

Raul (Age 43): I love this book, it's the real deal. The food plans are bomb, and I've got more energy for everything. I'm even getting compliments from the fam. Feels good!

Darnell (Age 46): Let me tell you, this book is a AMAZING. It's not just about losing weight; it's about feeling good in your own skin. The food is legit, and I'm making moves!

Luis (Age 40): This book is changing the game for me. It's got me thinking about food in a whole new way. The meals are fire, and I'm dropping pounds while still grubbing on good stuff.

Marcus (Age 42): This book is like my new best friend. It's teaching me how to eat better without being all complicated. I'm seeing results, and it's like a fresh start for my health.